The Delicious G Mediterranean I

A Complete Collection of Amazing Mediterranean Recipes to Boost Your Appetite and Satisfy Your Taste

Carl Ewing

Table of Contents

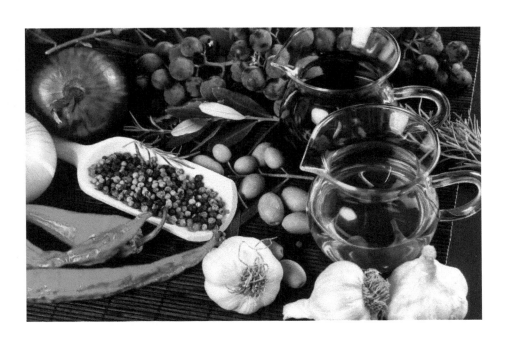

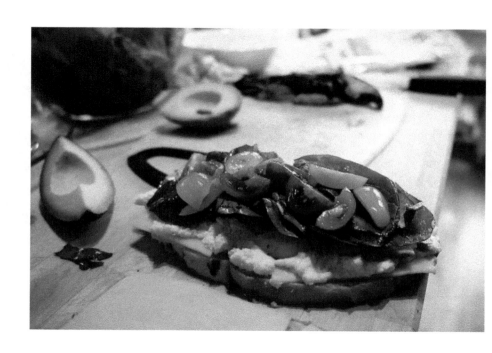

Coconut Beets

Prep time: 5 minutes I **Cooking time:** 20 minutes I

Servings: 4

Ingredients:

- 1 pound beets, peeled and cubed
- 1 red onion, chopped
- 1 tablespoon olive oil
- ½ cup coconut cream
- 4 tablespoons non-fat yogurt
- 1 tablespoon chives, chopped

Directions:

1. Heat up a pan with the oil over medium heat, add the onion, stir and sauté for 4 minutes.
2. Add the beets, cream and the other ingredients, toss, cook over medium heat for 15 minutes more, divide between plates and serve.

Nutrition facts per serving: calories 250, fat 13.4, fiber 3, carbs 13.3, protein 6.4

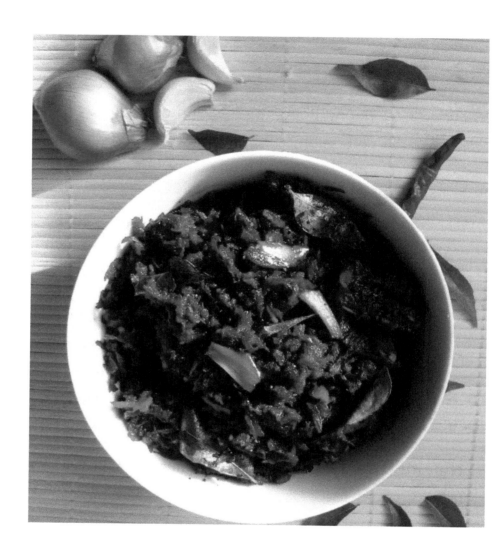

Avocado Mix

Prep time: 10 minutes I **Cooking time:** 14 minutes I

Servings: 4

Ingredients:

- 1 tablespoon avocado oil
- 1 teaspoon sweet paprika
- 1 pound mixed bell peppers, cut into strips
- 1 avocado, peeled, pitted and halved
- 1 teaspoon garlic powder
- 1 teaspoon rosemary, dried
- ½ cup veggie stock
- Black pepper to the taste

Directions:

1. Heat up a pan with the oil over medium-high heat, add all the bell peppers, stir and sauté for 5 minutes.
2. Add the rest of the ingredients, toss, cook for 9 minutes more over medium heat, divide between plates and serve.

Nutrition facts per serving: calories 245, fat 13.8, fiber 5, carbs 22.5, protein 5.4

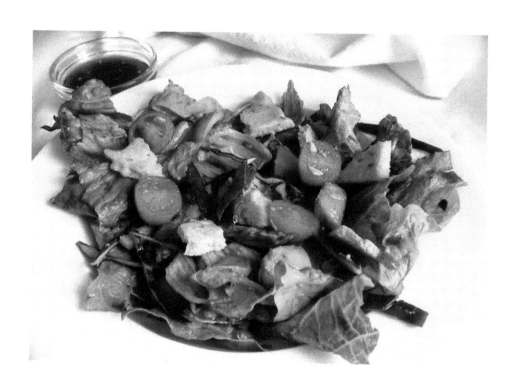

Roasted Sweet Potato

Prep time: 10 minutes I **Cooking time:** 1 hour I

Servings: 4

Ingredients:

- 3 tablespoons olive oil
- 2 sweet potatoes, peeled and cut into wedges
- 2 beets, peeled, and cut into wedges
- 1 tablespoon oregano, chopped
- 1 tablespoon lime juice
- Black pepper to the taste

Directions:

1. Arrange the sweet potatoes and the beets on a lined baking sheet, add the rest of the ingredients, toss, introduce in the oven and bake at 375 degrees F for 1 hour/
2. Divide between plates and serve as a side dish.

Nutrition facts per serving: calories 240, fat 11.2, fiber 4, carbs 8.6, protein 12.1

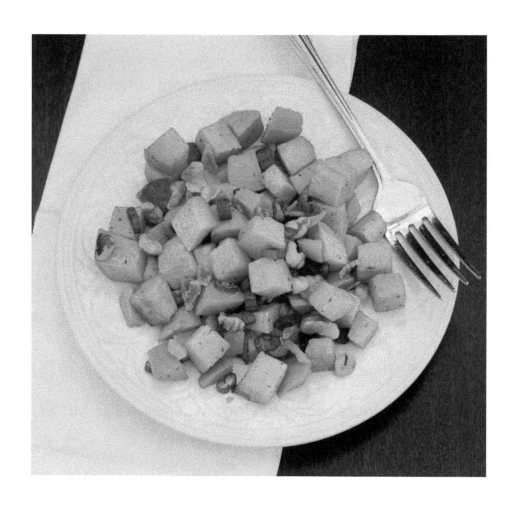

Coconut Kale Sauté

Prep time: 10 minutes I **Cooking time:** 15 minutes I

Servings: 4

Ingredients:

- 2 tablespoons olive oil
- 3 tablespoons coconut aminos
- 1 pound kale, torn
- 1 red onion, chopped
- 2 garlic cloves, minced
- 1 tablespoon lime juice
- 1 tablespoon cilantro, chopped

Directions:

1. Heat up a pan with the olive oil over medium heat, add the onion and the garlic and sauté for 5 minutes.
2. Add the kale and the other ingredients, toss, cook over medium heat for 10 minutes, divide between plates and serve.

Nutrition facts per serving: calories 200, fat 7.1, fiber 2, carbs 6.4, protein 6

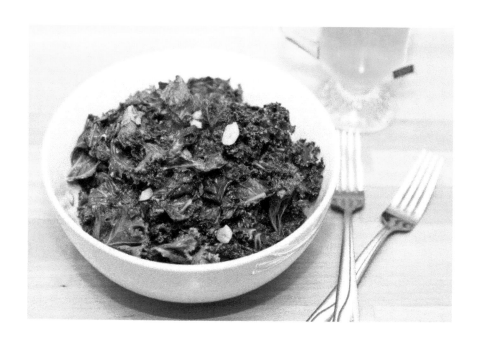

Allspice Carrots

Prep time: 10 minutes I **Cooking time:** 20 minutes I

Servings: 4

Ingredients:

- 1 tablespoon lemon juice
- 1 tablespoon olive oil
- ½ teaspoon allspice, ground
- ½ teaspoon cumin, ground
- ½ teaspoon nutmeg, ground
- 1 pound baby carrots, trimmed
- 1 tablespoon rosemary, chopped
- Black pepper to the taste

Directions:

1. In a roasting pan, combine the carrots with the lemon juice, oil and the other ingredients, toss, introduce in the oven and bake at 400 degrees F for 20 minutes.
2. Divide between plates and serve.

Nutrition facts per serving: calories 260, fat 11.2, fiber 4.5, carbs 8.3, protein 4.3

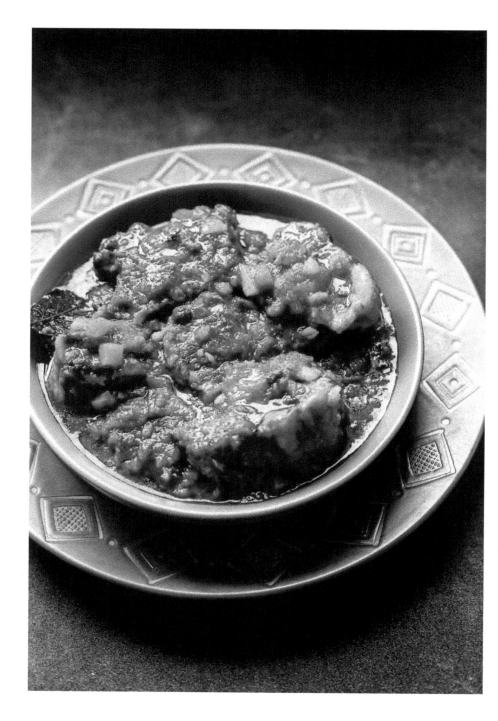

Lemony Dill Artichokes

Prep time: 10 minutes I **Cooking time:** 20 minutes I
Servings: 4

Ingredients:

- 2 tablespoons lemon juice
- 4 artichokes, trimmed and halved
- 1 tablespoon dill, chopped
- 2 tablespoons olive oil
- A pinch of black pepper

Directions:

1. In a roasting pan, combine the artichokes with the lemon juice and the other ingredients, toss gently and bake at 400 degrees F for 20 minutes.

   Divide between plates and serve.

Nutrition facts per serving: calories 140, fat 7.3, fiber 8.9, carbs 17.7, protein 5.5

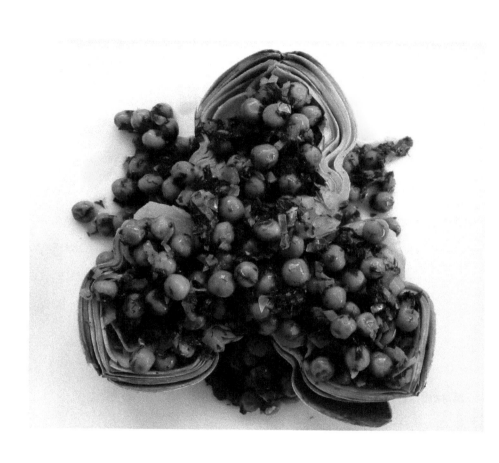

Veggie Chips

Prep time: 10 minutes I **Cooking time:** 30 minutes I

Servings: 4

Ingredients:

- 1 pound carrots, peeled and thinly sliced
- Salt and black pepper to the taste
- ½ teaspoon rosemary, dried
- 1 tablespoon chives, chopped
- Cooking spray

Directions:

1. Spray a baking sheet with cooking spray, spread the carrots chips, add the rest of the ingredients, toss and bake at 390 degrees F for 30 minutes.
2. Divide the chips into bowls and serve.

Nutrition facts per serving: calories 48, fat 0.2, fiber 2.9, carbs 11.3, protein 1

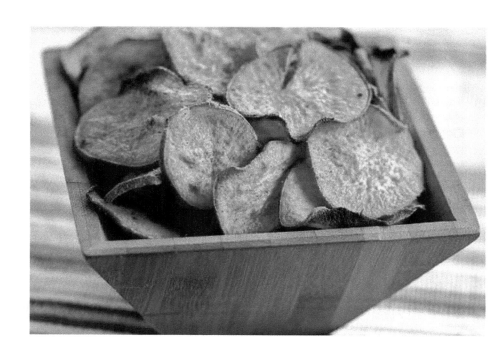

Rosemary Potato Wedges

Prep time: 10 minutes I **Cooking time:** 35 minutes I
Servings: 4

Ingredients:

- 2 sweet potatoes, peeled and cut into wedges
- Salt and black pepper to the taste
- 2 tablespoons olive oil
- 1 tablespoon rosemary, chopped
- 2 tablespoons balsamic vinegar

Directions:

1. Spread the potato wedges on a baking sheet lined with parchment paper, add the rest of the ingredients, toss and bake at 400 degrees F for 35 minutes.
2. Divide into bowls and serve as a snack.

Nutrition facts per serving: calories 153, fat 7.3, fiber 3.4, carbs 21.5, protein 1.2

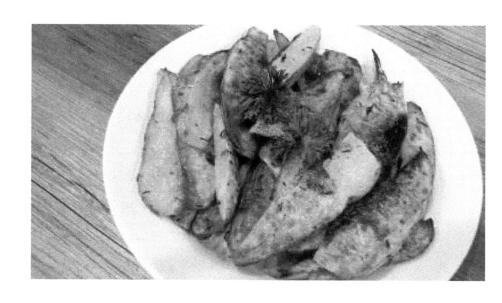

Spinach Dip

Prep time: 10 minutes I **Cooking time:** 20 minutes I

Servings: 5

Ingredients:

- 4 cups spinach, chopped
- 2 tablespoons olive oil
- Salt and black pepper to the taste
- 4 garlic cloves, minced
- ¾ cup tahini
- ½ cup coconut cream
- 1 tablespoon lime juice
- 1 tablespoon coriander, chopped

Directions:

1. Heat up a pan with the oil over medium heat, add the garlic and sauté for 2 minutes.
2. Add the spinach and the other ingredients, stir, cook for 18 minutes more, blend using an immersion blender, divide into bowls and serve.

Nutrition facts per serving: calories 408, fat 38.5, fiber 5.6, carbs 13.3, protein 9.4

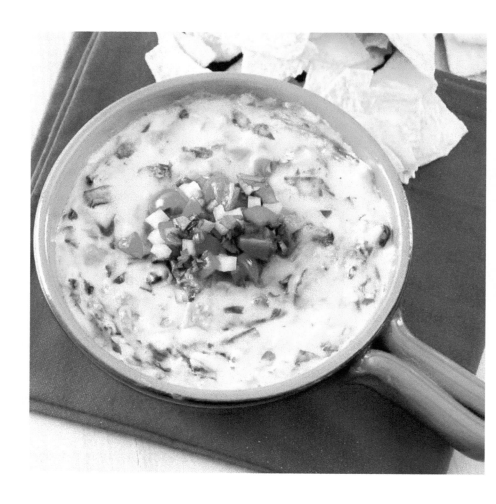

Avocado and Onion Spread

Prep time: 10 minutes I **Cooking time:** 0 minutes I

Servings: 6

Ingredients:

- 2 avocados, peeled and pitted
- 1 red onion, chopped
- 2 spring onions, chopped
- 1 tablespoon lemon juice
- 1 tablespoon cilantro, chopped
- A pinch of salt and black pepper

Directions:

1. Mash the avocados in a bowl, add the onion, the spring onions and the other ingredients, whisk and serve as a party dip.

Nutrition facts per serving: calories 219, fat 19.7, fiber 7.6, carbs 11.9, protein 2.4

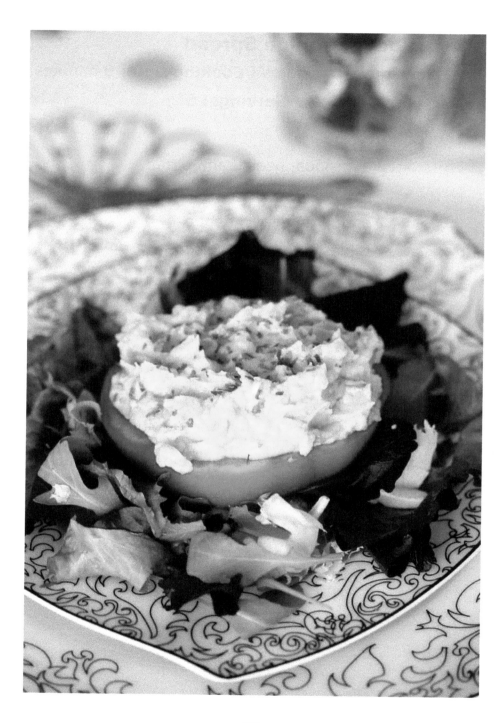

Curry Shrimp Appetizer

Prep time: 5 minutes I **Cooking time:** 10 minutes I

Servings: 4

Ingredients:

- 1 pound shrimp, peeled and deveined
- 2 tablespoons olive oil
- 2 spring onions, chopped
- A pinch of salt and black pepper
- ½ teaspoon cumin, ground
- ½ teaspoon rosemary, dried
- 1 teaspoon curry powder
- 2 tablespoons chives, chopped

Directions:

1. Heat up a pan with the oil over medium heat, add the spring onions and sauté for 2 minutes.
2. Add the shrimp and the other ingredients, toss, cook for 8 minutes, arrange on a platter and serve.

Nutrition facts per serving: calories 201, fat 9.1, fiber 0.5, carbs 2.9, protein 26.1

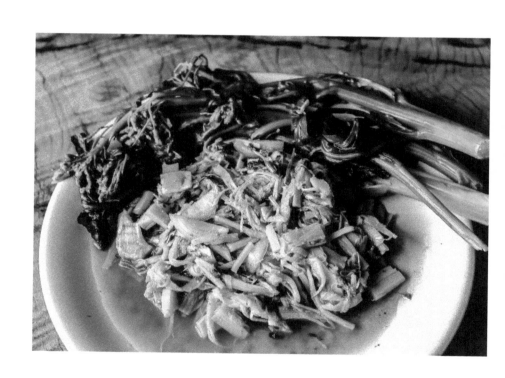

Pineapple and Tomato Salsa

Prep time: 10 minutes I **Cooking time:** 0 minutes I

Servings: 4

Ingredients:

- 2 cups pineapple, peeled and cubed
- 4 scallions, chopped
- ¼ cup cilantro, chopped
- 1 green chili pepper, chopped
- 2 tomatoes, cubed
- 2 tablespoons olive oil
- Salt and black pepper to the taste
- 1 tablespoon lemon juice
- A pinch cayenne pepper

Directions:

1. In a bowl, combine the pineapple with the scallions and the other ingredients, toss well and serve as a party salsa.

Nutrition facts per serving: calories 100, fat 3.8, fiber 4, carbs 8, protein 9

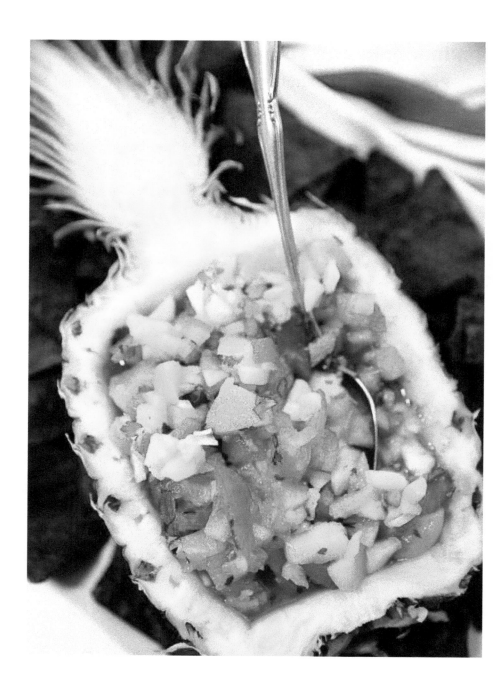

Italian Kale Dip

Prep time: 10 minutes I **Cooking time:** 30 minutes I

Servings: 6

Ingredients:

- 2 cups kale, chopped
- 1 yellow onion, chopped
- Salt and black pepper to the taste
- 2 tablespoons avocado oil
- Juice of 1 lemon
- 1 teaspoon Italian seasoning
- ¼ teaspoon chili powder
- 1 teaspoon cumin, ground
- 1 cup coconut cream

Directions:

1. Heat up a pan with the oil over medium heat, add the onion and sauté for 5 minutes.
2. Add the kale, the cream and the other ingredients, whisk, cook over medium heat for 25 minutes more, blend using an immersion blender, divide into bowls and serve as a party dip.

Nutrition facts per serving: calories 126, fat 7, fiber 2, carbs 9, protein 7

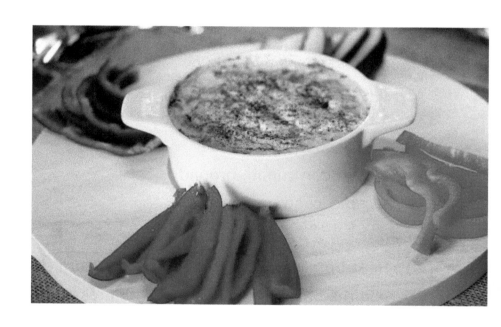

Coconut Dip

Prep time: 10 minutes I **Cooking time:** 20 minutes I

Servings: 8

Ingredients:

- 1 garlic head, peeled and cloves separated
- 1 cup coconut cream
- 1 cup spinach, torn
- 1 tablespoon olive oil
- 1 teaspoon rosemary, dried
- 1 tablespoon chives, chopped
- A pinch of salt and black pepper

Directions:

1. Heat up a pan with the oil over medium heat, add the garlic and sauté for 10 minutes.
2. Add the spinach, cream and the other ingredients, whisk, cook over medium heat for 10 minutes more, blend using an immersion blender, divide into bowls and serve.

Nutrition facts per serving: calories 100, fat 3, fiber 4, carbs 8, protein 5

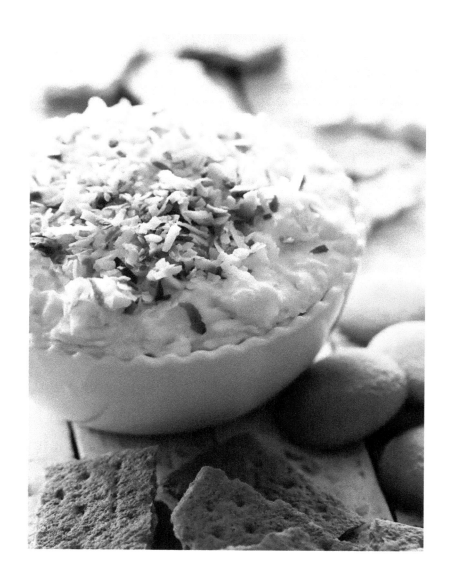

Tahini Peppers Spread

Prep time: 10 minutes I **Cooking time:** 0 minutes I

Servings: 6

Ingredients:

- 1 cup roasted red peppers, minced
- 1 tablespoon avocado oil
- 4 garlic cloves, chopped
- ½ cup tahini paste
- 2 tablespoons lemon juice
- 1 tablespoon cilantro, chopped
- A pinch of salt and black pepper

Directions:

1. In a blender, mix the peppers with the oil, the garlic and the other ingredients, pulse well, divide into bowls and serve as a party spread.

Nutrition facts per serving: calories 140, fat 6, fiber 2, carbs 9, protein 8

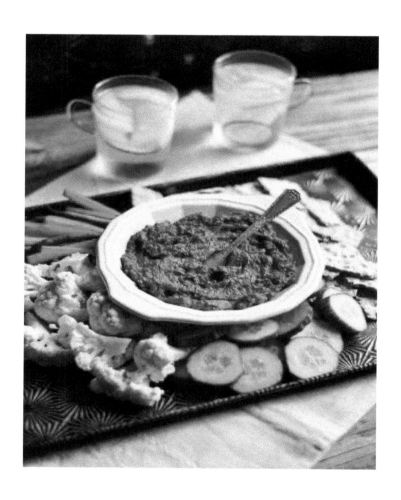

Turmeric Mushroom Spread

Prep time: 10 minutes I **Cooking time:** 25 minutes I

Servings: 8

Ingredients:

- 1 tablespoon olive oil
- 1 yellow onion, chopped
- 1 pound white mushrooms, sliced
- 1 teaspoon turmeric powder
- 1 teaspoon coriander, ground
- 3 garlic cloves, minced
- 2 cups coconut cream
- A pinch of salt and black pepper
- 1 tablespoon dill, chopped

Directions:

1. Heat up a pan with the oil over medium heat, add the onion and the garlic and sauté for 5 minutes.
2. Add the mushrooms and sauté for 5 minutes more.
3. Add the rest of the ingredients, stir, cook over medium heat for 15 minutes, blend using an immersion blender, divide into bowls and serve.

Nutrition facts per serving: calories 120, fat 8, fiber 5, carbs 10, protein 9

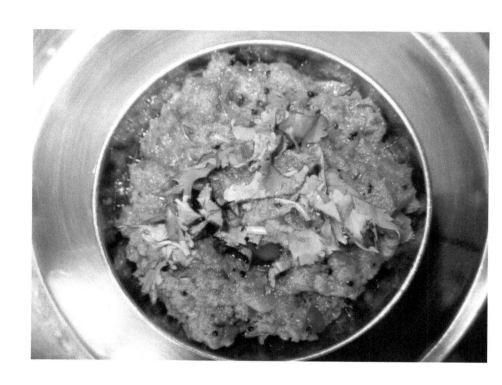

Lime Dip

Prep time: 10 minutes I **Cooking time:** 0 minutes I

Servings: 6

Ingredients:

- 1 cup coconut cream
- 2 tablespoons cilantro, chopped
- ½ cup baby spinach
- A pinch of salt and black pepper
- Juice of 1 lime
- ½ teaspoon cumin, ground
- 3 garlic cloves, chopped

Directions:

1. In your blender, combine the cream with the cilantro and the other ingredients, pulse, divide into bowls and serve as a party dip.

Nutrition facts per serving: calories 120, fat 12, fiber 2, carbs 11, protein 5

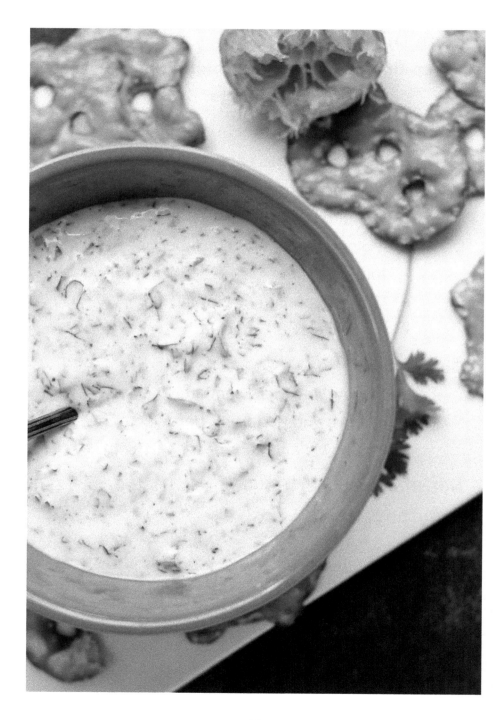

Lime Olives Dip

Prep time: 10 minutes I **Cooking time:** 0 minutes I

Servings: 8

Ingredients:

- 2 cups black olives, pitted and sliced
- A pinch of salt and black pepper
- 4 tablespoons olive oil
- 4 garlic cloves, chopped
- Juice of 1 lime
- 1 tablespoon cilantro, chopped

Directions:

1. In a blender, combine the olives with salt, pepper and the other ingredients, pulse well, divide into small bowls and serve as a party dip.

Nutrition facts per serving: calories 165, fat 11, fiber 4, carbs 8, protein 5

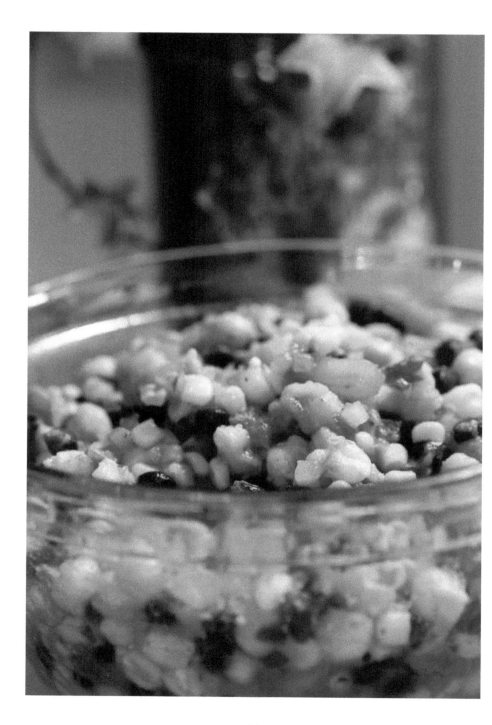

Coconut Bok Choy Dip

Prep time: 10 minutes I **Cooking time:** 25 minutes I

Servings: 6

Ingredients:

- 2 garlic cloves, minced
- 1 pound bok choy, torn
- 1 yellow onion, chopped
- 1 cup coconut cream
- 1 tablespoon olive oil
- 1 tablespoon cilantro, chopped
- A pinch of salt and black pepper

Directions:

1. Heat up a pan with the oil over medium heat, add the onion and the garlic and sauté for 5 minutes.
2. Add the rest of the ingredients, stir, cook over medium heat for 20 minutes, blend using an immersion blender, divide into bowls and serve.

Nutrition facts per serving: calories 150, fat 2, fiber 3, carbs 8, protein 5

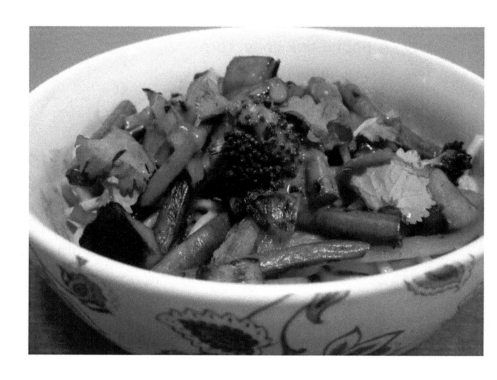

Walnuts Snack

Prep time: 10 minutes I **Cooking time:** 14 minutes I
Servings: 4

Ingredients:

- 1 cup walnuts
- 1 tablespoon olive oil
- 1 teaspoon garlic powder
- 1 teaspoon smoked paprika
- A pinch of salt and black pepper

Directions:

1. Spread the walnuts on a baking sheet lined with parchment paper, add the oil and the other ingredients, toss and bake at 400 degrees F for 14 minutes.
2. Divide the mix into bowls and serve.

Nutrition facts per serving: calories 100, fat 2, fiber 4, carbs 11, protein 6

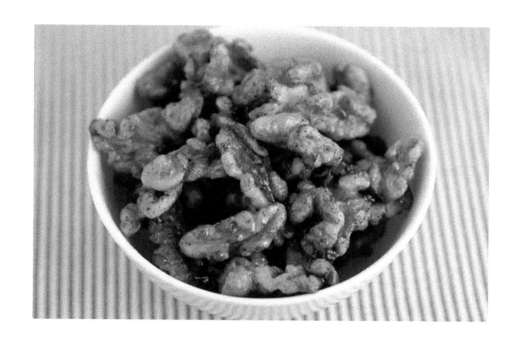

Lentils and Tomato Salsa

Prep time: 10 minutes I **Cooking time:** 20 minutes I
Servings: 8

Ingredients:

- 1 yellow onion, sliced
- 2 spring onions, chopped
- 1 cup cherry tomatoes, halved
- 1 cucumber, cubed
- 1 cup red lentils, cooked
- 1 tablespoon lemon juice
- ¼ cup parsley, chopped
- 1 tablespoon curry powder
- 1 tablespoon olive oil

Directions:

1. Heat up a pan with the oil over medium heat, add the onion and spring onions and sauté for 5 minutes.
2. Add the lentils and the other ingredients, toss, cook over medium heat for 15 minutes, divide into small bowls and serve cold.

Nutrition facts per serving: calories 142, fat 4, fiber 3, carbs 8, protein 8

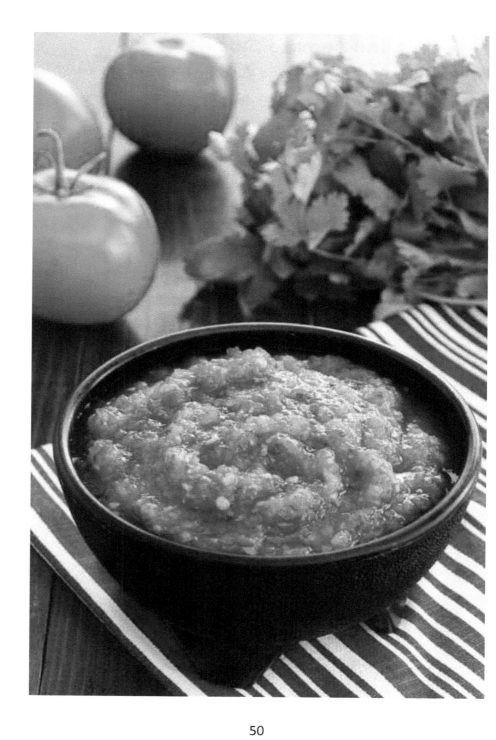

Garlic Tomato Salsa

Prep time: 10 minutes I **Cooking time:** 0 minutes I

Servings: 6

Ingredients:

- 1 pound cherry tomatoes, halved
- 1 cup zucchini, cut with a spiralizer
- 2 tablespoons olive oil
- 3 spring onions, chopped
- 3 garlic cloves, minced
- 2 teaspoons balsamic vinegar
- 1 tablespoon basil, chopped
- A pinch of salt and black pepper

Directions:

1. In a bowl, combine the tomatoes with the zucchinis and the other ingredients, toss well and serve.

Nutrition facts per serving: calories 121, fat 3, fiber 1, carbs 8, protein 6

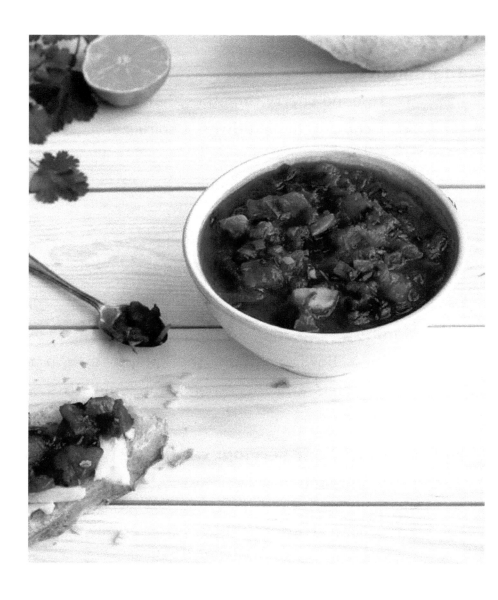

Masala Dip

Prep time: 10 minutes I **Cooking time:** 0 minutes I
Servings: 8

Ingredients:

- ½ cup walnuts, chopped
- 1 cup coconut cream
- ½ teaspoon chili powder
- A pinch of salt and black pepper
- ½ teaspoon garlic powder
- 1 teaspoon cumin, ground
- 1 teaspoon garam masala

Directions:

1. In a blender, combine the walnuts with the cream, the chili powder and the other ingredients, pulse well, divide into bowls and serve as a party dip.

Nutrition facts per serving: calories 152, fat 5, fiber 7, carbs 9, protein 8

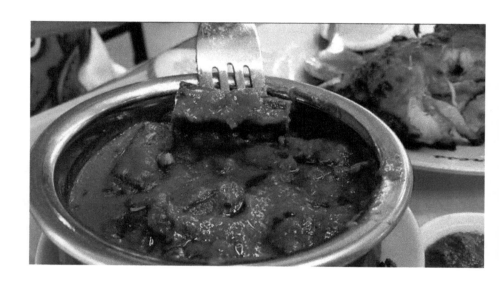

Sage Dip

Prep time: 10 minutes I **Cooking time:** 0 minutes I

Servings: 8

Ingredients:

- 1 cup spring onions, chopped
- 1 cup coconut cream
- 1 tablespoon tahini paste
- 1 tablespoon olive oil
- 1 teaspoon sage, ground
- A pinch of salt and black pepper

Directions:

1. In a blender, combine the spring onions with the cream, the tahini paste and the other ingredients, pulse well, divide into bowls and serve cold.

Nutrition facts per serving: calories 112, fat 5, fiber 2, carbs 8, protein 7

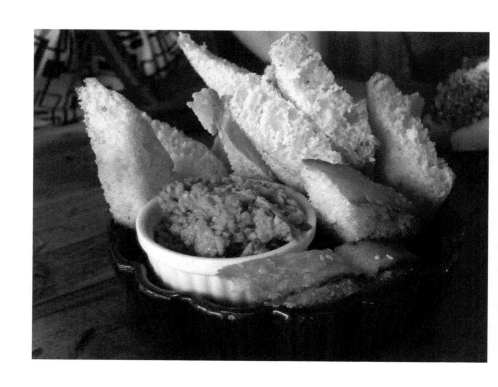

Broccoli Dip

Prep time: 10 minutes I **Cooking time:** 20 minutes I

Servings: 4

Ingredients:

- 1 pound broccoli florets
- 1 cup spinach leaves, torn
- 1 cup coconut cream
- 1 tablespoon olive oil
- 1 yellow onion, chopped
- A pinch of salt and black pepper
- 1 teaspoon smoked paprika
- ½ teaspoon chili powder
- ¼ teaspoon mustard powder

Directions:

1. Heat up a pan with the oil over medium heat, add the onion and sauté for 5 minutes.
2. Add the broccoli, the spinach and the other ingredients, stir, bring to a simmer and cook over medium heat for 15 minutes more.
3. Blend using an immersion blender, divide into bowls and serve.

Nutrition facts per serving: calories 223, fat 18.4, fiber 5.4, carbs 14.3, protein 5.2

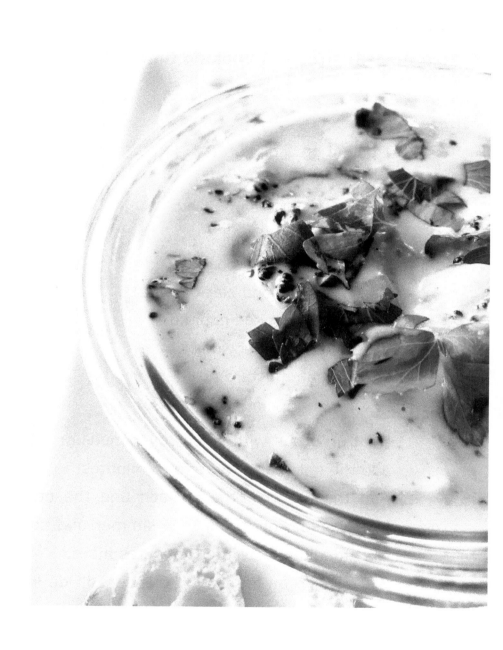

Coconut Chard Dip

Prep time: 5 minutes I **Cooking time:** 20 minutes I
Servings: 4

Ingredients:

- 2 cups chard leaves
- 1 cup coconut cream
- ¼ cup tahini paste
- 1 tablespoon olive oil
- 1 yellow onion, chopped
- 1 teaspoon chili powder
- 1 teaspoon sweet paprika
- A pinch of salt and black pepper
- Juice of 1 lime
- 1 tablespoon cilantro, chopped

Directions:

1. Heat up a pan with the oil over medium heat, add the onion, chili powder and the paprika, stir and cook for 5 minutes.
2. Add the chard and the other ingredients except the cream and the tahini paste, stir, cook over medium heat for 15 minutes more and transfer to a blender.
3. Add the remaining ingredients, pulse well, divide into bowls and serve as a party dip.

Nutrition facts per serving: calories 278, fat 26.1, fiber 4.1, carbs 11.4, protein 4.8

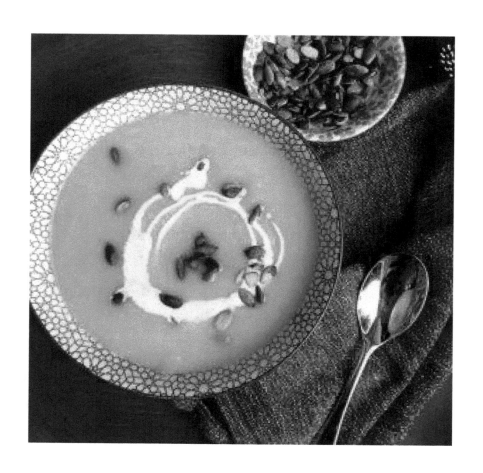

Paprika Seeds Snack

Prep time: 10 minutes I **Cooking time:** 15 minutes I

Servings: 4

Ingredients:

- ½ cup sunflower seeds
- ½ cup chia seeds
- ½ cup pine nuts
- ½ cup pumpkin seeds
- 1 tablespoon coconut oil, melted
- 1 teaspoon sweet paprika

Directions:

1. Spread the seeds on a baking sheet lined with parchment paper, add the oil and the paprika, toss and cook for 15 minutes at 400 degrees F.
2. Divide into bowls and serve.

Nutrition facts per serving: calories 110, fat 1, fiber 5, carbs 7, protein 5

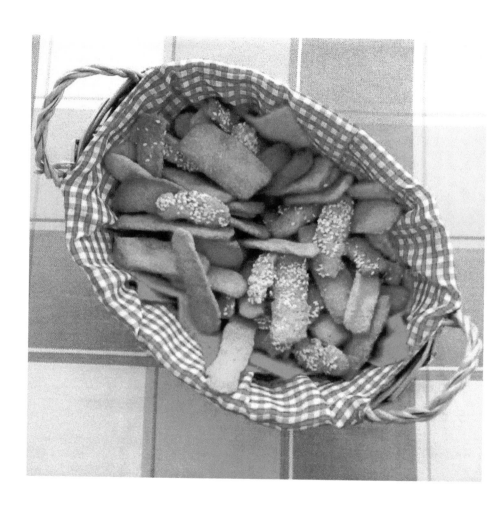

Peas Salsa

Prep time: 10 minutes I **Cooking time:** 0 minutes I

Servings: 4

Ingredients:

- 1 cup cherry tomatoes, halved
- 2 cups snow peas, steamed and cooled
- 1 tablespoon lemon juice
- 2 garlic cloves, minced
- 1 avocado, peeled, pitted and cubed
- 1 tablespoon olive oil
- 1 tablespoon cilantro, chopped
- A pinch of cayenne pepper

Directions:

1. In a bowl, mix the cherry tomatoes with the peas and the other ingredients, toss well, divide into smaller bowls and serve.

Nutrition facts per serving: calories 120, fat 2, fiber 4, carbs 6, protein 6

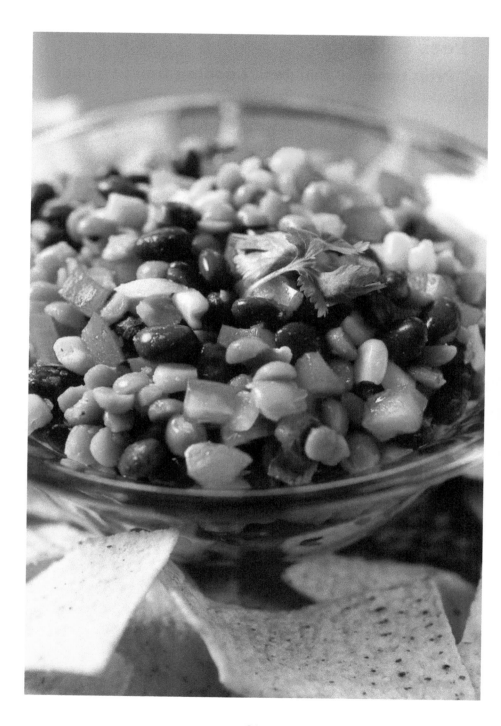

Nutmeg Apple Chips

Prep time: 10 minutes I **Cooking time:** 1 hour I

Servings: 4

Ingredients:

- Cooking spray
- 2 apples, cored thinly sliced
- 1 tablespoon cinnamon powder
- A pinch of nutmeg, ground

Directions:

1. Arrange the apples on a lined baking sheet, add the other ingredients, toss and cook at 360 degrees F for 1 hour.
2. Divide into bowls and serve as a snack

Nutrition facts per serving: calories 141, fat 2, fiber 2, carbs 7, protein 5

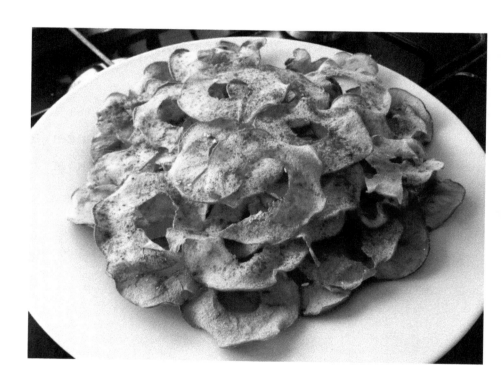

Cucumber Spread

Prep time: 10 minutes I **Cooking time:** 0 minutes I

Servings: 4

Ingredients:

- 2 cups coconut cream
- 2 cucumbers, chopped
- 1 tablespoon dill, chopped
- 2 teaspoons thyme, dried
- 2 teaspoons parsley, dried
- 2 teaspoons chives, chopped
- A pinch of sea salt and black pepper

Directions:

1. In a blender, combine the cream with the cucumbers and the other ingredients, pulse, divide into bowls and serve cold.

Nutrition facts per serving: calories 120, fat 3, fiber 5, carbs 5, protein 3

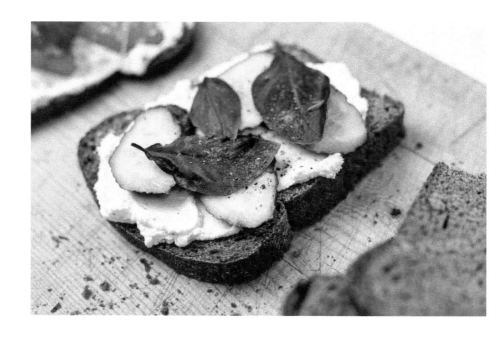

Beans, Cucumber and Tomato Salsa

Prep time: 15 minutes I **Cooking time:** 0 minutes I

Servings: 6

Ingredients:

- 1 cup garbanzo beans, cooked
- 1 cup black beans, cooked
- ½ cup cherry tomatoes, cubed
- 1 cucumber, cubed
- 2 tablespoons lime juice
- 1 tablespoon olive oil
- 5 garlic cloves, minced
- ½ teaspoon cumin, ground
- A pinch of salt and black pepper

Directions:

1. In a bowl, combine the beans with the tomatoes, cucumber and the other ingredients, toss well and serve cold as a snack.

Nutrition facts per serving: calories 170, fat 3, fiber 7, carbs 10, protein 8

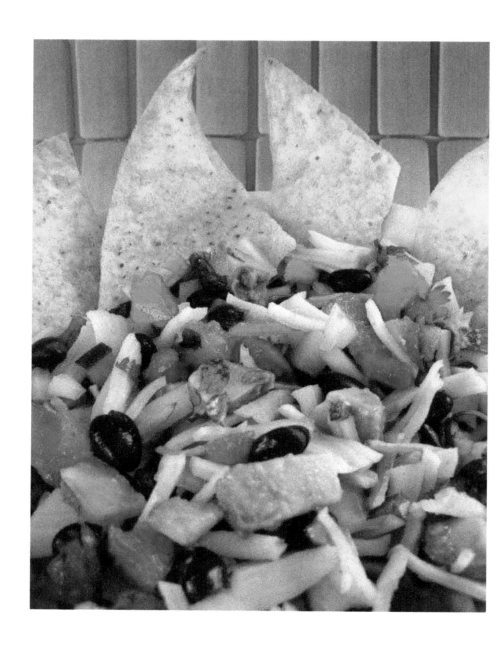

Bell Peppers Cakes

Prep time: 10 minutes I **Cooking time:** 10 minutes I

Servings: 6

Ingredients:

- 1 tablespoon olive oil
- ½ cup cilantro, chopped
- 2 spring onions, chopped
- 1 red bell pepper, chopped
- 1 green bell pepper, chopped
- 1 egg
- ½ cup almond flour
- A pinch of salt and black pepper
- 2 garlic cloves, minced
- 3 zucchinis, grated

Directions:

1. In a bowl, combine the zucchinis with the bell peppers and the other ingredients except the oil, stir well and shape medium patties out of this mix.
2. Heat up a pan with the oil over medium heat, add the patties, cook for 5 minutes on each side, arrange on a platter and serve.

Nutrition facts per serving: calories 120, fat 4, fiber 2, carbs 6, protein 6

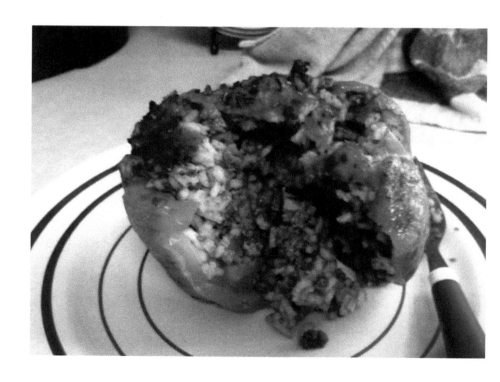

Italian Broccoli Bowls

Prep time: 10 minutes I **Cooking time:** 25 minutes I
Servings: 4

Ingredients:

- 1 pound broccoli florets
- Cooking spray
- 2 eggs, whisked
- 1 teaspoon Italian seasoning
- A pinch of sea salt and black pepper
- 1 teaspoon smoked paprika
- 1 teaspoon cumin, ground

Directions:

1. In a bowl, mix the eggs with the Italian seasoning and the other ingredients except the broccoli and the cooking spray and whisk well.

2. Dip the broccoli florets in the eggs mix, arrange them on a baking sheet lined with parchment paper, grease them with cooking spray and bake at 380 degrees F for 25 minutes.

3. Divide the broccoli bites into bowls and serve.

Nutrition facts per serving: calories 120, fat 6, fiber 2, carbs 6, protein 7

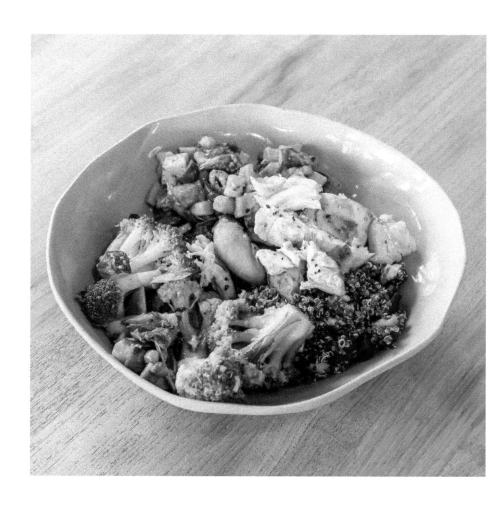

Mushrooms Bowls

Prep time: 10 minutes I **Cooking time:** 25 minutes I

Servings: 6

Ingredients:

- 2 pound brown mushroom caps
- 1 tablespoon olive oil
- A pinch of sea salt and black pepper
- 1 tablespoon balsamic vinegar
- 1 tablespoon chives, chopped
- 1 teaspoon sweet paprika

Directions:

1. Arrange mushroom caps on a baking sheet lined with parchment paper, add the oil, salt, pepper and the other ingredients, toss well and bake at 390 degrees F for 25 minutes.
2. Divide the mushroom caps in bowls and serve.

Nutrition facts per serving: calories 120, fat 2, fiber 2, carbs 6, protein 5

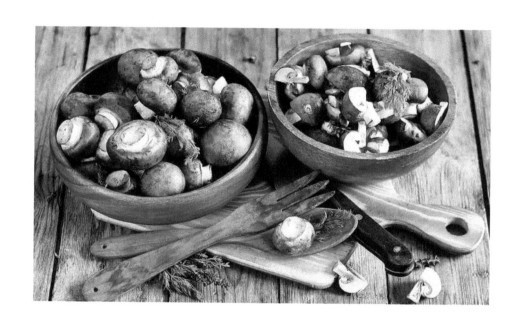

Artichoke Spread

Prep time: 10 minutes I **Cooking time:** 35 minutes I

Servings: 8

Ingredients:

- ½ cup almond milk
- 1 cup coconut cream
- 10 ounces artichoke hearts, chopped
- 4 garlic cloves, minced
- A pinch of black pepper
- 1 tablespoon oregano, dried

Directions:

1. In a pan, combine the cream with the almond milk and the other ingredients, toss, bring to a simmer and cook over medium heat for 35 minutes.
2. Blend the mix using an immersion blender, divide into bowls and serve as a party dip.

Nutrition facts per serving: calories 130, fat 5, fiber 4, carbs 6, protein 6

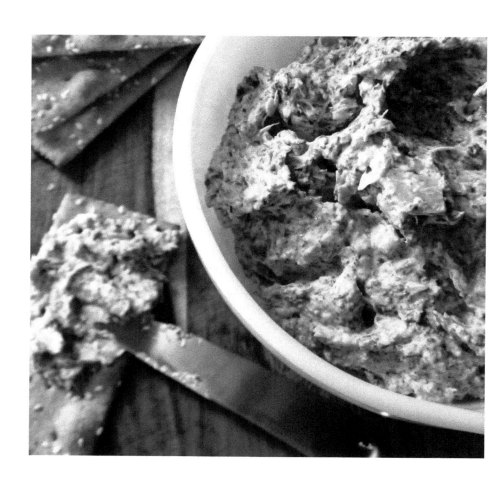

Ginger Pineapple Snack

Prep time: 10 minutes I **Cooking time:** 20 minutes I

Servings: 6

Ingredients:

- 14 ounces pineapple, cubed
- ½ teaspoon ginger, grated
- 1 tablespoon balsamic vinegar
- ½ teaspoon rosemary, dried
- 1 tablespoon olive oil

Directions:

1. In a bowl, combine the pineapple bites with the ginger and the other ingredients, toss, divide into bowls and serve as a snack.

Nutrition facts per serving: calories 54, fat 2.4, fiber 1, carbs 8.9, protein 0.4

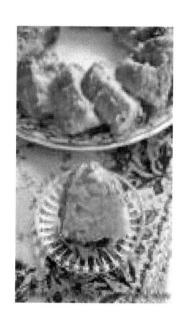

Onions Bowls

Prep time: 10 minutes I **Cooking time:** 12 minutes I

Servings: 4

Ingredients:

- 2 cups pearl onions, peeled
- Juice of 1 lime
- 1 tablespoon olive oil
- 1 tablespoon ginger, grated
- 1 teaspoon turmeric powder
- 1 small parsley bunch, chopped
- A pinch of salt and black pepper

Directions:

1. Heat up a pan with the oil over medium-high heat, add the pearl onions, lime juice and the other ingredients, toss and cook over medium heat for 12 minutes.
2. Divide the mix into bowls and serve as a snack.

Nutrition facts per serving: calories 135, fat 2, fiber 4, carbs 9, protein 12

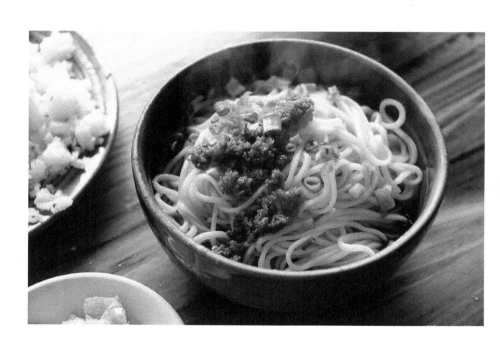

Ginger Clams

Prep time: 10 minutes I **Cooking time:** 12 minutes I

Servings: 4

Ingredients:

- 1 pound clams, scrubbed
- 3 garlic cloves, minced
- 1 tablespoon olive oil
- 1 teaspoon ginger, grated
- 1 teaspoon chili powder
- A pinch of sweet paprika
- ½ cup chicken stock

Directions:

1. Heat up a pan with the oil over medium heat, add the garlic and the ginger and sauté for 2 minutes.
2. Add the clams and the other ingredients, toss, bring to a simmer and cook over medium heat for 10 minutes.
3. Arrange the clams on a platter and serve.

Nutrition facts per serving: calories 93, fat 4, fiber 0.8, carbs 14, protein 1

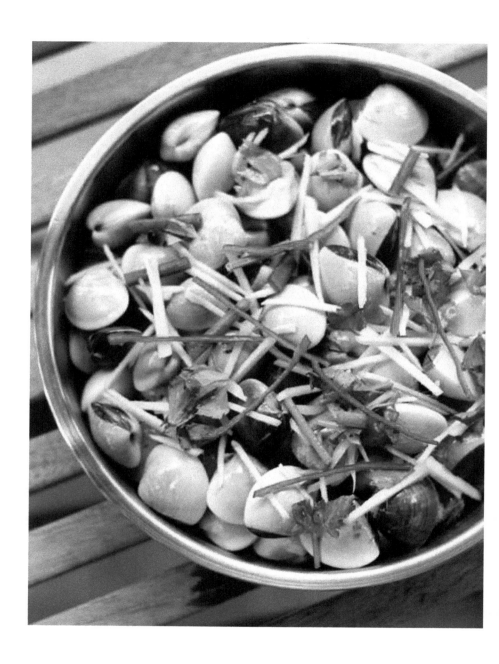

Dill Tuna Bites

Prep time: 10 minutes I **Cooking time:** 12 minutes I
Servings: 6

Ingredients:

- 1 pound tuna fillets, boneless and cut into cubes
- 2 teaspoons dill, chopped
- 2 tablespoons olive oil
- 1 teaspoon garlic powder
- Salt and black pepper to the taste
- 2 tablespoon chives, chopped
- 1 tablespoon mustard

Directions:

1. In a bowl, mix the tuna with the dill, oil and the other ingredients except the chives, toss well and arrange on a baking sheet lined with parchment paper.
2. Bake the tuna bites at 400 degrees F for 12 minutes, divide into small bowls, sprinkle the chives on top and serve.

Nutrition facts per serving: calories 140, fat 2, fiber 5, carbs 7, protein 6

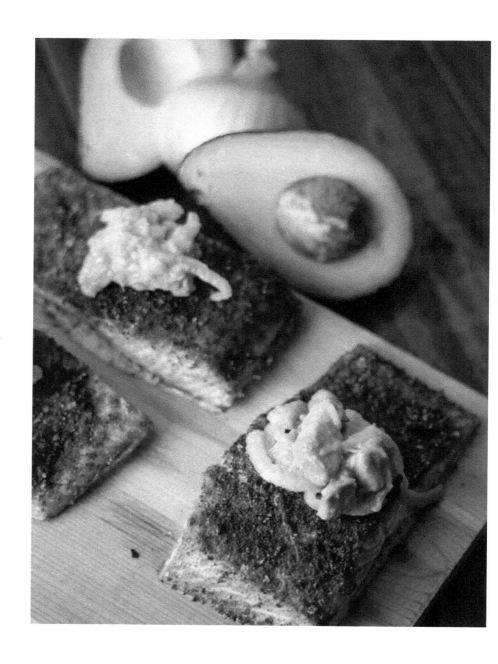

Green Chips

Prep time: 10 minutes I **Cooking time:** 15 minutes I
Servings: 4

Ingredients:

- 2 tablespoons olive oil
- 1 pound kale leaves, pat dried
- 2 tablespoons garlic, minced
- 1 tablespoon lemon zest, grated
- Salt and black pepper to the taste

Directions:

1. Spread the kale leaves on a baking sheet lined with parchment paper, add the oil and the other ingredients, toss a bit and cook in the oven at 400 degrees F for 15 minutes.
2. Cool the kale chips down, divide into bowls and serve as a snack.

Nutrition facts per serving: calories 149, fat 4, fiber 3, carbs 9, protein 6

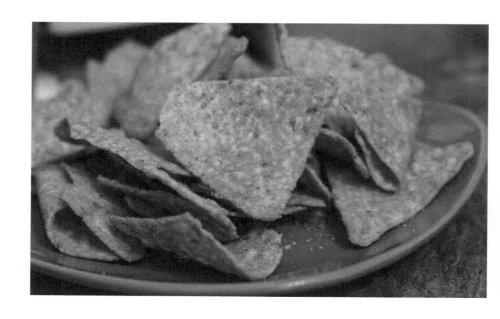

Peppers and Cilantro Salsa

Prep time: 10 minutes I **Cooking time:** 0 minutes I

Servings: 4

Ingredients:

- 1 pound mixed bell peppers, cut into strips
- 1 cup cherry tomatoes, cubed
- 1 cucumber, cubed
- 1 avocado, peeled, pitted and cubed
- Salt and black pepper to the taste
- 1 tablespoon olive oil
- ½ cup cilantro, chopped
- 1 tablespoon garlic, minced
- ½ cup green onion, chopped
- 1 tablespoon lemon juice

Directions:

1. In a bowl, combine the bell peppers with the tomatoes, cucumber, the avocado and the other ingredients, toss well, divide into small bowls and serve cold as a snack.

Nutrition facts per serving: calories 170, fat 13.6, fiber 5.1, carbs 12.8, protein 2.6

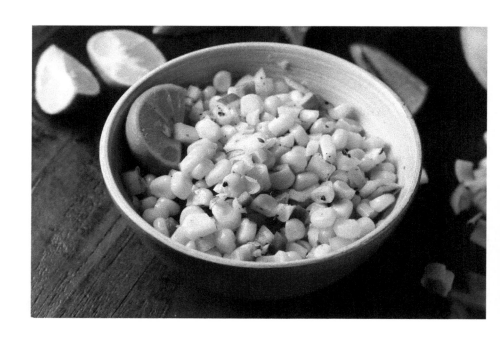

Shrimp Bowls

Prep time: 10 minutes

Cooking time: 0 minutes

Servings: 4

Ingredients:

- 1 pound shrimp, peeled, deveined, and cooked
- 1 cup kalamata olives, pitted and sliced
- 1 cup cherry tomatoes, cubed
- ½ cup basil, chopped
- A pinch of salt and black pepper
- 2 tablespoons lime juice
- 2 teaspoons chili powder

Directions:

1. In a bowl, combine the shrimp with the kalamata, tomatoes and the other ingredients, toss well, divide into smaller bowls and serve.

Nutrition facts per serving: calories 186, fat 5.8, fiber 2.1, carbs 6.4, protein 26.8

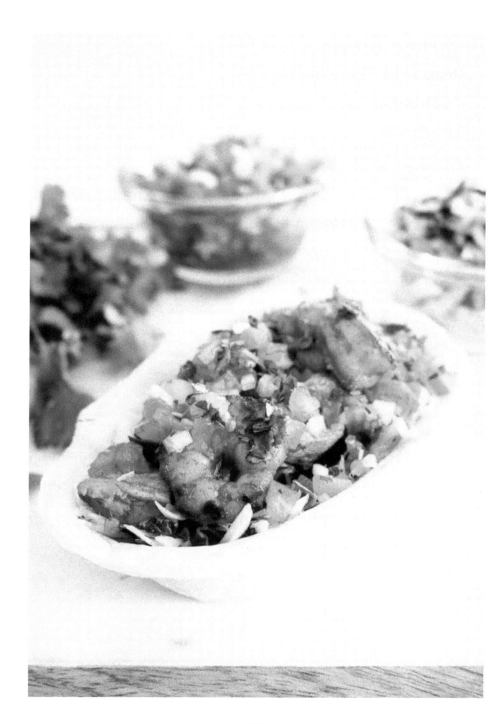

Italian Salmon Bowls

Prep time: 10 minutes I **Cooking time:** 14 minutes I

Servings: 4

Ingredients:

- 1 pound salmon fillets, boneless and cubed
- 2 tablespoons olive oil
- 1 teaspoon Italian seasoning
- 1 teaspoon garlic, minced
- ½ cup kalamata olives, pitted and chopped
- ¼ cup basil, chopped
- Salt and black pepper to the taste

Directions:

1. In a bowl, combine the salmon with the oil, the Italian seasoning and the other ingredients, toss, arrange on a baking sheet lined with parchment paper and cook at 400 degrees F for 14 minutes.
2. Divide the salmon into bowls and serve.

Nutrition facts per serving: calories 270, fat 7.5, fiber 2, carbs 7, protein 7

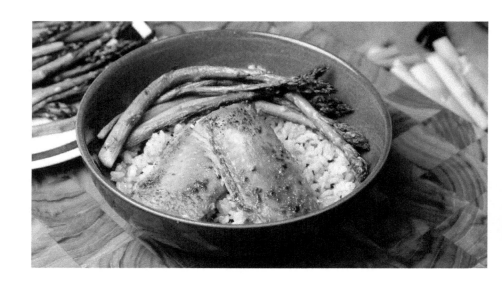

Avocado and Olives Salsa

Prep time: 10 minutes I **Cooking time:** 0 minutes I **Servings:** 4

Ingredients:

- 2 avocados, peeled, pitted and roughly cubed
- 2 tablespoons olive oil
- 1 cup kalamata olives, pitted and halved
- ½ cup cherry tomatoes, cubed
- Juice of 1 lime
- Salt and black pepper to the taste
- 1 tablespoon basil, chopped

Directions:

1. In a bowl, combine the avocados with the lime juice and the other ingredients, toss, divide into small bowls and serve as a snack.

Nutrition facts per serving: calories 180, fat 3, fiber 5, carbs 8, protein 6

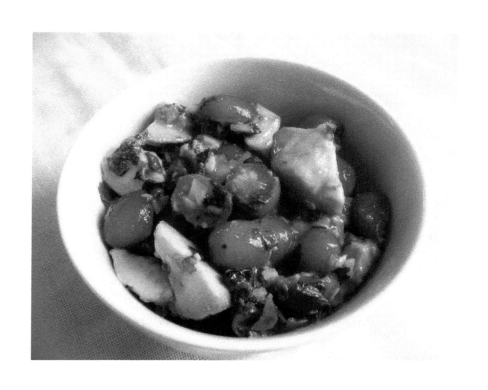

Seafood Bowls

Prep time: 5 minutes I **Cooking time:** 10 minutes I
Servings: 4

Ingredients:

- 1 pound mussels, debearded and scrubbed
- ½ pound shrimp, peeled and deveined
- 4 scallions, chopped
- 2 garlic cloves, minced
- 1 tablespoon olive oil
- 1 tablespoon lemon juice

Directions:

1. Heat up a pan with the oil over medium heat, add the scallions and the garlic and sauté for 2 minutes.
2. Add the rest of the ingredients, toss, cook over medium heat for 8 minutes more, divide into bowls and serve.

Nutrition facts per serving: calories 90, fat 4, fiber 5, carbs 5, protein 2

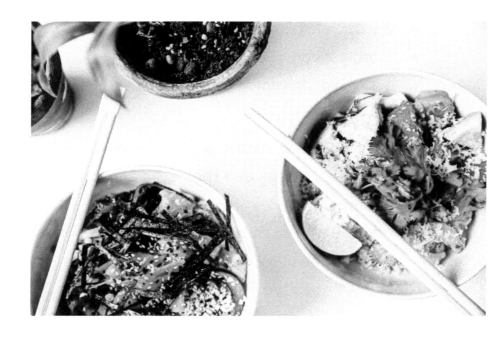

Cayenne Calamari Bites

Prep time: 10 minutes I **Cooking time:** 20 minutes I

Servings: 4

Ingredients:

- 1 pound calamari rings
- 2 tablespoons olive oil
- ½ cup chicken stock
- A pinch of cayenne pepper
- A pinch of salt and black pepper
- 1 tablespoons lemon juice
- 1 teaspoon chili powder
- 1 teaspoon cumin, ground
- 1 tablespoon chives, chopped

Directions:

1. Heat up a pan with the oil over medium heat, add the calamari, the stock and the other ingredients, toss, cook for 20 minutes, divide into small bowls and serve.

Nutrition facts per serving: calories 155, fat 8, fiber 3, carbs 3, protein 7

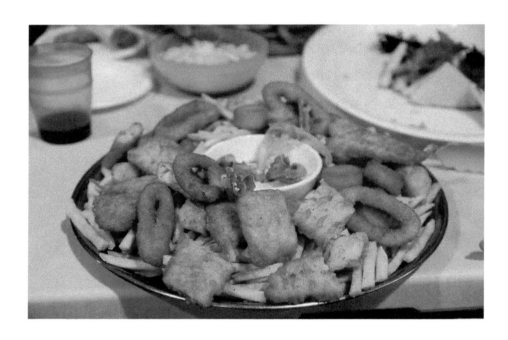

Turmeric Seafood Mix

Prep time: 10 minutes I **Cooking time:** 12 minutes I

Servings: 4

Ingredients:

- 1 cup calamari rings
- 1 cup clams, scrubbed
- 1 pound shrimp, peeled and deveined
- 1 tablespoon avocado oil
- 1 teaspoon lemon juice
- ½ teaspoon rosemary, dried
- 1 teaspoon chili powder
- ½ cup chicken stock
- Salt and black pepper to the taste
- ½ teaspoon turmeric powder

Directions:

1. Heat up a pan with the oil over medium heat, add the shrimp, the calamari rings, the clams and the other ingredients, toss, cook for 12 minutes, arrange on a platter and serve.

Nutrition facts per serving: calories 238, fat 8, fiber 3, carbs 10, protein 8

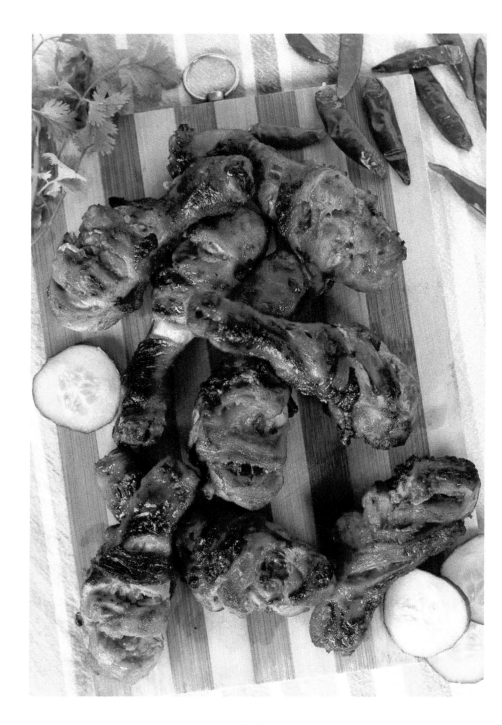

Coconut Celery Spread

Prep time: 10 minutes I **Cooking time:** 15 minutes I
Servings: 4

Ingredients:

- 4 celery stalks
- 3 scallions, chopped
- 1 tablespoon olive oil
- 1 tablespoon lime juice
- ½ teaspoon chili powder
- 1 cup coconut cream
- Salt and black pepper to the taste
- 2 tablespoons parsley, chopped

Directions:

1. Heat up a pan with the oil over medium heat, add the scallions and sauté for 2 minutes.
2. Add the celery and the other ingredients, toss, cook over medium heat for 13 minutes more, blend using an immersion blender, divide into bowls and serve s a snack.

Nutrition facts per serving: calories 140, fat 10, fiber 3, carbs 6, protein 13

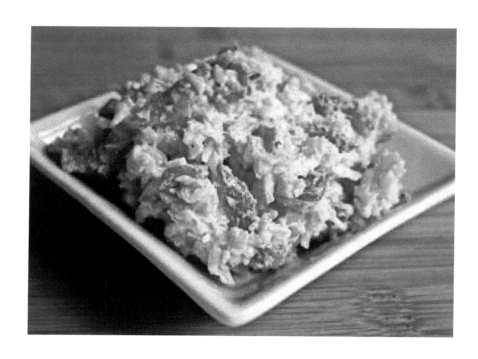

Creamy Coconut Shrimp

Prep time: 5 minutes I **Cooking time:** 10 minutes I

Servings: 4

Ingredients:

- 1 pound shrimp, peeled and deveined
- 2 shallots, chopped
- 1 tablespoon olive oil
- Salt and black pepper to the taste
- 1 teaspoon rosemary, dried
- 2 cups coconut cream
- 1 cup cilantro, chopped

Directions:

1. Heat up a pan with the oil over medium heat, add the shallots and sauté for 2 minutes.
2. Add the shrimp and the other ingredients, toss, cook over medium heat for 8 minutes, divide into bowls and serve.

Nutrition facts per serving: calories 220, fat 8, fiber 0, carbs 5, protein 12

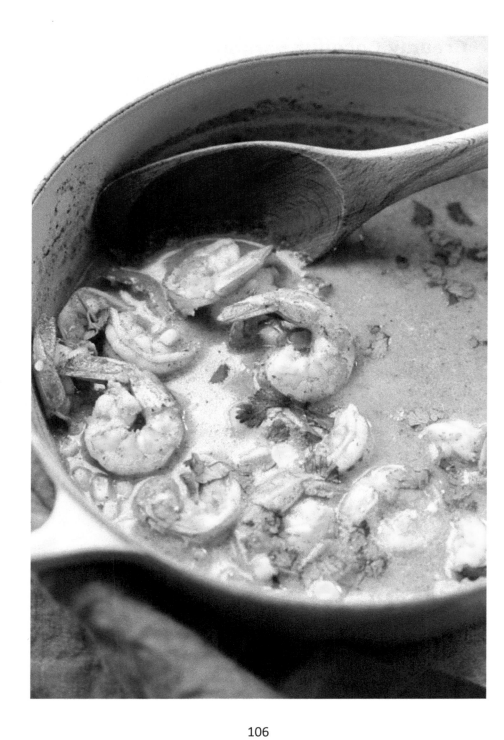

Herbed Salsa

Prep time: 10 minutes I **Cooking time:** 0 minutes I
Servings: 4

Ingredients:

- 2 tablespoons olive oil
- 2 fennel bulbs, shredded
- 1 cup kalamata olives, pitted and halved
- 1 tablespoon balsamic vinegar
- A pinch of salt and black pepper
- 2 tablespoons lime juice
- 2 tablespoons parsley, chopped
- 2 tablespoons mint, chopped

Directions:

1. In a bowl, mix the fennel with the oil and the other ingredients, toss well, keep in the fridge for 10 minutes, divide into bowls and serve.

Nutrition facts per serving: calories 160, fat 7, fiber 2, carbs 7, protein 8

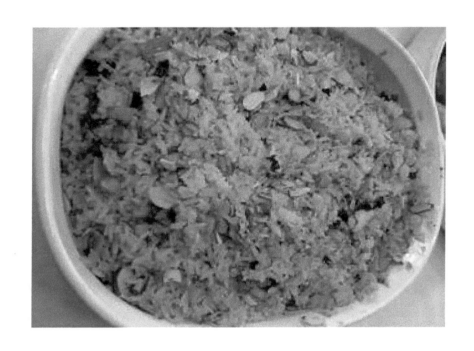

Mango Salsa

Prep time: 10 minutes I **Cooking time:** 0 minutes I
Servings: 4

Ingredients:

- 2 mangoes, peeled and cubed
- 2 oranges, peeled and cut into segments
- ½ cup kalamata olives, pitted and halved
- Juice of 1 orange
- Zest of 1 orange, grated
- Juice of 1 lime
- 2 red chili peppers, chopped
- ½ teaspoon ginger, grated
- A pinch of salt and black pepper
- 1 tablespoon avocado oil
- ¼ cup cilantro, chopped

Directions:

1. In a bowl, mix the mangoes with the oranges and the other ingredients, toss, divide into smaller bowls and serve.

Nutrition facts per serving: calories 170, fat 3, fiber 5.7, carbs 37.6, protein 2.5

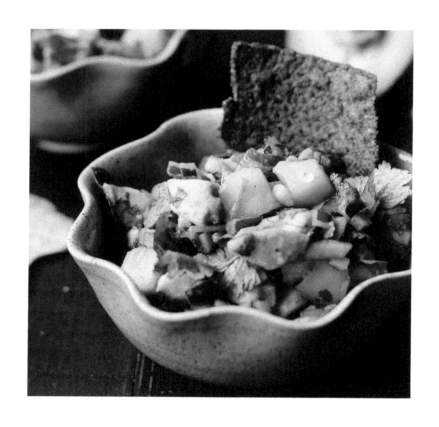

Lightning Source UK Ltd.
Milton Keynes UK
UKHW020813180621
385734UK00005B/118